UNEVEN
SURFACES

VICTORIA PONTE

Printed in the United States of America
First Printing 2020
First Edition 2020

10 9 8 7 6 5 4 3 2 1

For My Mom and Dad and the millions living with disabilities who understand what it means to navigate uneven surfaces.

Table of Contents

Foreword

This book is a collection of essays written over the course of 21 years since I had a stroke on February 14, 1999 when I was 35 and 6 months pregnant with my second son. It is my hope that this memoir will be a survival guide of sorts for anyone going through a life altering traumatic experience and has the will to persevere to living their best life after surviving it. I hope it inspires you to live your life with gratitude, wonder and a sense of humor.

PART I

What Happened, The Beginning

Chapter 1

Uneven Surfaces

I was learning how to walk for the second time in my life. I was 35 years old. I had recently given birth to my second son.

A sudden severe stroke in the 26th week of pregnancy had left me totally paralyzed on the left half of my body.

I spent 53 days in bed, pregnant and paralyzed, waiting to give birth so I could be moved to a rehabilitation hospital.

I gave birth in the usual way while I was still hemiplegic. 4 days later, I was taken in an ambulance to an inpatient rehabilitation hospital. I had no idea how long I would be there. I was extremely weak, depressed, spastic, and in chronic pain.

I would spend six hours a day in physical, occupational and speech therapy. We worked on building strength and learning to walk in physical therapy.

We worked on "activities of daily living" such as getting dressed in occupational therapy. Speech therapy centered around cognitive exercises to improve things such as executive functioning, a term to describe planning how to execute everyday tasks in steps. My ability to speak and understand was not affected.

My left foot remained paralyzed as I regained movement in my arm and leg. I was fitted for a brace to keep my foot lifted while I was learning to walk. I used a cane for help with my disrupted sense of balance.

I never imagined walking could be so difficult. My left arm spastically flailed each time I took a step further impairing my sense of balance.

I made progress and was soon walking around the smooth, level, tile floors of the hospital. The entire facility was on one level, but we worked on going up and down a set of wooden steps in the physical therapy room.

Just as I was feeling comfortable walking, the therapists decided to take me outside to the "therapeutic garden." The simple act of stepping outside the hospital for the first time in weeks really threw me for a loop. Gone were the smooth, level floors.

The garden was a small patch of grass and sand with steps to take you to different levels. When I stepped on the sand for the first time, I was sure I couldn't do this.

With support from 2 physical therapists, I walked the garden. It was scary and challenging for sure. The exercise in the therapeutic garden prepared me for years of adapting to life with half my body not working properly. As we figure out how to walk on a level surface, the floor beneath our feet constantly changes and we must adapt and keep walking.

Chapter 2

I Felt Helpless When I Had A Baby

It was a sudden loss of function of one hand but the baby came anyway expecting me to feed and diaper him, I thought it was impossible, and it was, but there were times when I refused to be so crippled, when I wrestled him up onto the table, and using the other hand I cleaned him up.

I remembered changing the first baby using both hands. Now there was injustice. Sadness. Anger and frustration along with the joy of motherhood. It was a joy to nurse him.

But there were too many things I couldn't do this time. I mostly sat in the wheelchair and watched.

Other people taking care of my babies. Felt like I was an imposter in my own home.

Too many things were different with the second baby. And he grew up anyway.

Chapter 3
My Dog Died From a Broken Heart

I thought all I wanted was my dog. I was pregnant, paralyzed and confined to a hospital bed for 53 days.

Barney was my first "baby." He was an 8 week old golden retriever when he became part of the family.

My sister got permission from the hospital to bring him to the entrance of the hospital and to bring me outside in my wheelchair to "walk" him. I had been gone a month.

Barney was happy to see me and clearly very nervous. I was not the same after the surgery.

I held his leash with my only functioning hand. In his excitement and fear, he ran through the sidewalks around the hospital and down the road in back.

I was so happy to see him, but it certainly didn't feel like I was "walking" him.

My husband was a bit cagey when he told me Barney was sick. He didn't elaborate over the course of quite a few visits to see me in the hospital.

Barney was never the same after I had the stroke. I returned home 3 months later in a wheelchair. I was never the same, either.

My husband finally told me Barney had leukemia after I got home. He had been trying to protect me from the sad news while I was in the hospital for 3 months.

I watched him decline and get sicker at home. When he finally had to be euthanized 6 months later, I was unable to get on the ground with him as he lay bleeding. I couldn't travel to the vet with him for his final car ride, either.

It felt like the cause of death was really heartbreak because Barney had   lost   *me*   6   months   earlier.

Chapter 4
This Is How I Found Out I Had A Stroke

I remembered I was pregnant when I woke up. I recognized all of my visitors. I understood I was in the hospital. I was able to have conversations with my family and friends.

What I couldn't figure out was how I got there. I didn't understand why the hair was shaved off half of my head. Or why my scalp was stapled.

I didn't know why the left half of my body felt as if it had been filled with cement, or why I was unable to move it. My left arm was bent and pressing hard on my 6 months pregnant belly on its own volition.

This was all happening after I was awakened from a 2 weeks long, medically induced coma. I was 35 years old, and had a husband and 22 month old son at home.

I remembered the last time I had walked around shopping for furniture for the new baby's room. Now I couldn't walk at all.

I had so many questions. My family explained that I'd had an AVM, or arteriovenous malformation in my brain.

They went on to explain that an AVM is a tangled mass of blood vessels that was likely present since birth. In my case, the only symptom came on the day it ruptured, February 14, 1999. I woke up with a severe headache and unable to move half of my body.

I had no memory of this happening or of being taken to the hospital in an ambulance. I don't remember having the CAT scan that determined my brain was bleeding after the doctors saw my pupils were fixed and dilated in the emergency room.

I struggled to make sense of my predicament. I was a strong, healthy young woman and suddenly I was an invalid in the hospital.

The story of the tangled mass of blood vessels rupturing possibly because of the extra blood volume of pregnancy stressing it made some sense. But it was still hard to accept that I was going to have a baby while I was paralyzed with little hope of being able to take care of the baby on my own. As the weeks passed, it was clear I would not be going home for some time.

I lied in bed, pregnant and paralyzed, for 7 weeks. I delivered the baby in the usual way while I was still hemiplegic with the help of nurses pushing on my paralyzed left side.

I was put in an ambulance and taken to a rehabilitation hospital 5 days after the baby was born in order to learn how to walk and take care of myself.

It was the strangest thing to go on a ride without being able to see where we were going. It looked like we were near a farm when I was taken out of the ambulance and taken inside in a wheelchair. The physical therapists who saw me first told me and my family that I was extremely weak and would need an unknown number of weeks of therapy before I was strong enough to go home. I spent about 8 hours a day in physical, occupational, and speech therapy. Progress was slow, but steady.

My age and condition prior to the hemorrhage helped.

I was lucky to have family nearby who visited me every day. My parents brought the new baby to the hospital every day so I could nurse him. Almost all the patients at the rehab hospital were elderly. I met one woman who had fallen and hit her head on New Year's Eve and was still there in April. She was close to my age and had young children.

My sister was sitting with me in the dining room one day for lunch where I was sitting with three much older women.

Everyone in the hospital was enchanted by the new baby who came to visit me every day. When I started explaining to the women at my table what happened to me by explaining about the tangled mass of blood vessels rupturing, a woman of about 75 or 80 said, "Just tell people you had a stroke." She seemed angry and annoyed that I had such a long explanation for what could have been explained in four simple words.

It was the first time I heard the word "stroke" to describe the rupture. I was a bit shocked. I thought strokes were something that happened to old people.

I went on to learn that any disruption of blood flow to the brain whether it's a hemorrhage or a blood clot is a stroke and can strike anyone at any time.

Chapter 5
I Didn't Want To Die, But Wished I Had

Through my depression after I had a stroke at age 35 while I was 6 months pregnant, my psychiatrist often asked me if I ever thought about ending my life. The depression came from a powerful mix of organic causes (a brain injury), being postpartum, and massively difficult life circumstances.

I truly never thought about committing suicide even when I was in a wheelchair with a 2 year old son and a newborn. But, I did have moments of wishing I had died in the emergency room or on the operating table during the brain surgery that saved my life. Even if my family would have suffered a crushing loss, I would be dead and not be feeling much.

The recovery and rehabilitation that were necessary because the left side of my body was completely paralyzed after surgery was brutal. There was constant chronic pain along with a body that would not cooperate. I spent six weeks in a rehabilitation hospital while my newborn son stayed with my parents. I had to relearn how to walk and take care of myself. I had some issues with executive functioning where I had to learn how to think about planning actions to accomplish everyday tasks.

Life at home was not the return to normal I had hoped for, but instead was a depressing, difficult battle to try to build some kind of life that resembled the old one. It was 7 months before I could return to driving. I relied on hired help to care for my two babies. I couldn't enjoy any of my old hobbies except for reading because of the loss of motor control. My husband became disengaged. This went on for years. Progress was very slow. But I was grateful to be alive as I knew that most people who have hemorrhagic strokes do not survive. And the ones that do are often not able to walk, speak, drive and otherwise enjoy life at all. The baby I was carrying was born healthy and was thriving.

I worked very hard at maintaining an attitude of gratitude. Every doctor I saw helped me understand how lucky I was.

With no end in sight to the struggle I was living with, I couldn't help but occasionally feel I would have been better off dead. It would have been easier for me, but terribly worse for my family. When I heard the news this year of Luke Perry's death at age 52 following 2 strokes, my first thought was he was lucky he didn't survive and have to go through what I did.

It's been 21 years since I had the stroke. My life has steadily improved even if I'm still living with chronic pain and a movement disorder. I haven't thought I wished I had died from it since those first five years of my recovery. I have become immensely better at being happy to just be alive and grateful for all the blessings in my life.

Chapter 6
Touched

Sometime after undergoing a lifesaving craniotomy, I read an explanation of the origin of the word "touched" to mean insane or crazy. It reputedly came from the idea that if your brain has been "touched" you are never right or the same again. Fortunately, most of our brains are never touched.

My brain was hemorrhaging due to a congenital defect. Had it continued untouched, I would have certainly died. A highly skilled neurosurgeon drilled a hole in my skull and used a saw to cut a circle out so he could access the part that was bleeding and clean it up. I have a horseshoe shaped scar under the mass of curly hair on my head.

I made a dramatic recovery from the surgery. I always maintained that I was "still me" as I could not perceive myself as others did from outside of my own head. I had some awareness of changes in my thinking and personality mostly from what others told me.

Most changes were physical. The damage to my brain resulted in serious motor control issues on my left side. To say it was a gargantuan adjustment to living with this wouldn't begin to describe it.

I once saw a very experienced psychotherapist about how to deal with the massive changes in my life. When I told her my husband continually told me I was not the same, and he had a hard time dealing with it, her response was "Of course you're not the same, you're better". This was a few years after the surgery and I was thriving in the face of horrible circumstances.

I was definitely touched. I won't deny that having to adjust to becoming disabled during my second pregnancy when I was a 35 year old mother of a two year old may have made me a little insane.

PART II

Fallout: What Happened Next

Chapter 7
Mother's Day Tea

My firstborn son, Sam, was in kindergarten and brought home an adorable, handmade invitation to a "Mother's Day Tea." It said it was an event for the moms and grandmothers of the entire kindergarten class, but each student was limited to 2 guests which in Sam's case would mean excluding 1 grandmother.

Both of his grandmothers had been very involved in his care since I had a disabling stroke when he was 22 months old, and gave birth to his brother just before he turned 2. It was not an easy decision to exclude my mother and invite my mother in law instead. Sam had spent a great deal of time at his "Oma's" when his dad was at work and I was in the hospital for 3 months. My mother in law was not one of my biggest fans, having married her favorite, firstborn son. She was crazy about Sam, though. My mother had been to a few events in Sam's class and didn't mind giving Oma a turn.

We lived in a tony suburb of New York City in one of the country's wealthiest zip codes. I had a hard time fitting in among the Stepford type wives who were married to the captains of industry, or were highly educated professionals in their own right. They were well-groomed, physically fit, fashionable and drove fine cars which they garaged in their interior decorator appointed McMansions.

I had been physically challenged since Sam was 22 months old. I wore a brace on my leg that needed to be worn in orthopedic shoes, carried a cane, limped and had a spastic left arm which kept me from carrying treats into the school like the other moms did effortlessly. I did manage to make some friends among the women at school, but never quite fit in and was more self-conscious in a school setting than I was when I wasn't around the other fancy moms who were ubiquitous.

I was a bit nervous about attending the Mother's Day Tea party, but I was sure I couldn't miss it for anything. I had developed an attitude of gratitude for my life and limited abilities to participate and enjoy it. I was certain I had survived the stroke against the odds for the purpose of being a mother to my two sons. I knew I was lucky to be alive and able to enjoy days like this.

I'm sure I looked nice because it wasn't as if I didn't have any good clothes to wear. It was a big day for my mother in law, too, because she was not very social in her own right.

The classroom was decorated with pastel colored spring flowers made from construction paper and paste. There were a series of low tables pushed together with paper plate place settings. The small chairs were a challenge.

Our children put on a special Mother's Day musical performance, and served the moms tea and cookies.

At the conclusion of the show, each child was asked to read out loud a story they had written about what made their mom special and why they loved her.

Sam was toward the end of the line and I listened intently to the other children's stories, all the while wondering what Sam was going to say. There were so many things I couldn't do that the other Moms were loved for. The children said things like: "I love you because you bake cookies for me."

"I love you because you take me to the park and play with me." "I love you because you play Legos with me."

"I love you because you read to me." "I love you because you love me."

"I love you because you make macaroni and cheese for me." About 20 kids said such cute things, and the suspense grew as they went down the linc to Sam. There were plenty of "oohs" and "ah" responses from the audience of mothers and grandmothers. Finally, it was Sam's turn. He said:

"I love you because you're beautiful."

There were a few seconds of silence as the room digested this perfectly sweet and original sentiment. Now I felt special among the group not because I was so physically different but because I was so proud of myself for bringing such an exceptional child up to kindergarten in the face of incredibly challenging circumstances.

Not one of the other children had said this about their mother. I was completely unaware that he saw me this way. My heart exploded with love and pride. My mother in law was impressed, as well.

Chapter 8

Both Of My Sons Had The Exact Same Mother, Only
Different

Their birthdays are 10 days apart. Two years, and 10 days. They have the same father. 2 boys. Somehow we expect our children to be similar. There are usually some similarities, and often drastic differences. Due to very unforeseen circumstances my sons each had a very different mother. And of course, their personalities and dispositions diverge quite a bit.

When I had my first son, Travis, in 1997, I was 32 years old. I was a fit and trim athlete before I became pregnant. I had protracted fertility struggles and lost 3 pregnancies prior to having my first full term pregnancy. I was over the moon when I gave birth.

I decided to be a stay at home mom for Travis and enjoy every minute of it. I breastfed him for 15 months. I took him for swimming lessons when he was 7 months old. I put him in a backpack and went hiking. I made friends with a woman at Gymboree when he was 6 months old and we did everything together. Her daughter was a day older than Travis. We also went to music classes together. I remember that first year as one of the best of my life.

My husband and I wanted 2 children. After our fertility struggles we decided it would be wise to not wait too long before trying for another. Ben was conceived the old fashioned way within 6 months. I was thrilled to think I was going to be able to do it all again with a new human. This time I had to have more tests during pregnancy due to my "advanced maternal age". Everything was fine.

That winter, my husband planned a ski weekend over Valentine's Day. I didn't think it was that important that we do something together because I never cared much about Valentine's Day one way or the other. As the day approached, he started to feel guilty about leaving me home alone and cancelled his plans.

My husband is a terrible snorer so I often slept in the guest bedroom that we were going to convert to the baby's room.

On the morning of Valentine's Day, my husband remembers waking up and thinking his biggest problem was going to be where to get me flowers. I woke up alone in the guestroom. I don't remember much until days later but my husband told me I was complaining of a splitting headache and called for help. I couldn't get up but I was awake. I peed the bed. It was the first day Travis climbed out of his crib. He was 22 months old. It wasn't long before my husband figured out it was a medical emergency and called 911.

The ambulance arrived quickly very early on an extremely cold February morning in New Jersey. The EMT's asked my husband if it would be ok for them to carry me down the stairs in a body bag because a stretcher might be dangerous with my pregnant size. They didn't zipper the bag up over my face. I had a seizure and passed out.

A CAT scan at the hospital revealed an extremely large cerebral hemorrhage. My pupils were fixed and dilated which indicated my brain stem functions such as respiration were shutting down. I was 26 weeks pregnant.

An emergency craniotomy saved our lives. The obstetrician scrubbed in for the surgery in case an emergency C section became necessary. The neurosurgeon opened my skull and cleaned up the bleeding mess in my brain. It went well.

I was put in a medically induced coma for recovery so my head would be as still as possible for 2 weeks. The entire left side of my body was completely paralyzed. My left arm was bent and locked in position pressing on my pregnant belly from spasticity. Nurses monitored the baby several times per day.

When I woke up, I was confused about why my body wasn't working. I was aware of bandages on my head and drainage tubes coming out either side. I didn't know what happened. I seemed oddly unconcerned about being pregnant. It wasn't until much later that I realized I had had a stroke. They told me I had a tangled mass of blood vessels in my brain that had ruptured. I didn't realize that when your brain bleeds it's a stroke.

I had limited physical therapy in the hospital. Rehab facilities are not equipped to handle a pregnancy so they wouldn't admit me until after I gave birth. So with a team of very nervous physical therapists I got out of bed and started walking around the halls of the hospital.

The plan was to leave the baby as long as possible so the lungs could fully develop. We assumed they would do a C section. I went into labor a few times but it was arrested with drugs. I was throwing up all the time and couldn't move.

On April 3rd, labor started again. This time, the drugs didn't stop its progression. I was still hemiplegic, but I delivered a healthy, 5 lb. 6 oz. boy in the usual way with a lot of help from nurses.

I was moved to a rehab hospital a few days later. I had lain in the acute care hospital, pregnant and paralyzed, for 53 days. My parents took the baby home with them so my husband could focus on taking care of Travis. We hired a baby nurse to help my parents with the late night feedings.

Our families rallied around to help. I learned how to walk again and take care of myself in rehab. I stayed there for six weeks all the while thinking everything would be fine when I went home. My arm was painfully spastic and nearly impossible to use. I became depressed from a combination of being postpartum, brain injured and living through horrible circumstances.

I went home in May in a wheelchair. We hired nannies to take care of my 6 week old and 2 year old babies.

It was a long, slow painful incomplete recovery. My sons had the same father. Travis had a very different mother than Ben. I won't know how Ben was affected by never knowing his mother as an able bodied person. Travis was definitely traumatized by the whole ordeal before he was verbal and able to talk about it. They have grown up to be very different individuals which I suppose happens under   any   circumstances.

Chapter 9
The Best Job I Ever Had

No pay, very little stress and a lot of fun. As part of my refusal to let my disability hinder my commitment to being the best mom I could for my kids, I volunteered to work at the school library when each of them were in kindergarten through third grade. I wasn't sure when I signed up if the physical demands would be too much for me, but I took the chance and was very glad I did.

I knew that I would mostly be seated at the desk where the students came to check out books. I was good at sitting and knew how to use a computer. I had some concern about not having the use of my left hand to do the job, but I knew I would figure it out as I had everything else in life over five years of becoming disabled eight weeks before my youngest son was born.

The librarian was a professional woman who had worked at the school for a long portion of her career. She took her job seriously and was dedicated. Mrs. M. was fascinated by the story of how I became disabled by a stroke while I was pregnant with my younger son. She made an effort to accommodate me by asking the other volunteers to shelve the books that were returned so I could sit at the desk and check out books because of my limited mobility.

It was sort of exciting for my kids to see me go to "work", since I had been disabled for their entire lives. It was a way for me to be like the other moms at school. I loved to watch them proudly tell their friends, "That's my mom." as they filed into the library with their class.

Mrs. M. had years of experience with unruly kids in the library. It is difficult for them to be quiet and listen. I sat at the desk and observed her call out and discipline many a five or six year old kid who just couldn't follow the library rules. Sometimes it was one of my own sons.

I loved meeting all of my kid's classmates. They were required to borrow a book every week. Sometimes the computer would tell me that a child had one or more books that were overdue. We usually wouldn't loan them another book in this case, but Mrs. M. kept track of just about every kid in the school and made carefully considered exceptions. She would know if there was any trouble in a particular child's home such as illness or divorce which would make keeping track of library books completely unimportant. I heard many adorable stories and excuses to my questions, "Do you have this book at home still? It was due two weeks ago." There is nothing like a five year old running through their train of thought out loud. "Well, I think it's still under my bed, I was going to bring it back, we didn't read it yet, can I still take out this book?" I was able to watch all of those kids grow up along with mine through high school graduation. I have an uncanny ability to remember names so they felt like I knew them when I greeted them by name around town or school.

There was a section of the library devoted to books for early readers where the younger students were encouraged to browse. Sometimes the kids got lost and would show up at the desk and ask to check out a 300 page novel. I would try to tactfully suggest they find another book, and offer to help them find one.

The best complaint I ever heard about a book was from a six year old who told me she didn't like it because it had "too many words." Working at the elementary school library was not paid employment, but I reaped rewards from those six years of volunteering that I have never seen in any paid job.

Chapter 10

If Your Children Are Pushing Your Buttons, Be Grateful

It felt like the one millionth trip to the orthodontist when my sons were in braces at the same time. It was a full time job chauffeuring them around suburbia when they were 11 and 13 years old. Doctor, dentist, psychologist, friends, school, repeat.

11 year old had an appointment after school one day so after picking them both up at the bus stop which is 1/4 mile from our house I had one errand to run at the shopping center then we had to go.

I was getting in the car when 13 year old starts begging for a sandwich from Subway on the other side of the parking lot. I firmly told him no because it would make us late, but he took off at a full run. I am not able to run at all or even walk normally. Yelling was no help. I know when I am defeated. I drove over to get him at the sandwich shop, then on to the orthodontist. I don't recall if we were late. I do remember being furious with him at first for being able to outrun me.

As I was driving on, I calmed down with the knowledge that I am fortunate to be the one the Universe chose to become disabled instead of my sons. I have seen many children with disabilities over the years in clinics and therapeutic settings. I was always grateful to be there for myself and not my kids.

My son had the intelligence, will and ability to execute a defiant plan to get what he wanted. I never forgot that day or stopped appreciating my kid's ability to defy me.

Chapter 11

They Always Had Nice Coats

We had a newborn son, as well as a two year old son. I was in a wheelchair. Looking back 21 years, I have trouble remembering how we did it. Raising children is the toughest job on the planet. Disable one parent, and the challenges multiply exponentially. I can remember days when I thought there was no way we could do it. In response, my mother always told me, "They will grow up anyway." That holds true no matter what your challenges may be. Time marches on. Our sons are now 21 and 23. Fortunately, I recovered enough from the crippling stroke to be able to be a good mother. I relearned how to walk, drive, cook and take care of myself. We were lucky to be able to afford hired help for the first four years of the newborn's life. Yet, on many levels, I was not an active mother.

I watched videos last weekend from our sons' early years. It seemed as if every moment of baby #1's life was unique. Each move was well documented. This is common among new parents.

Your first baby is the first one in the world to burp, poop, smile and laugh. I was physically fit for his first two years, and was seen carrying him, playing with him, and taking care of him.

Since I was six months pregnant with my second baby when I had the stroke, the scenes from his early life were mostly missing from the archive. It was not the same joyful, happy time after he was born. Much of the video footage consisted of my husband following the kids around with the camera while narrating the story. He was a good dad. They went on hikes, swam in the ocean, played in the snow, went ice skating on the lake at our place there, and fought physical battles like many brothers do. I wasn't able to participate in any of this. There was limited footage of me reading Curious George books to them on the couch. Sometimes I was passing through the scenes limping along. I attended their school plays and musical performances.

I watched these movies with amazement at what a beautiful time my kids seemed to have. They looked happy most of the time. I couldn't remember how we managed to dress them in such nice clothes. Where did we get the super nice, warm coats they wore with their mittens, hats and boots? Childhood passes in a blur no matter the circumstances. We were in survival mode for five years after our second baby was born. They grew up anyway.

Chapter 12

Graduation

I spent four years trying to act like I was like all of the other Moms. Still, so much of my identity was tied to the fact I was disabled. I felt the need to explain to everyone I met why I limped and carried a cane as a young woman. I assumed I looked so impaired it was what people were wondering about when they met me. At the end of the four years, I found out maybe my disability wasn't as glaring as I thought.

It seemed when I introduced myself to the moms I met at my son's preschool, I would always say something like, "My name is Victoria and I had a stroke while I was pregnant with my son who is in your child's class." People said some interesting things in response such as "You're kidding!" When they realized it definitely was not a joke, they were aghast.

Many were quite freaked out to hear that I had been 35 years old, 26 weeks pregnant, had a two year old, and woke up one day completely paralyzed on my left side. I was just like them except for this major fact.

We all had two year olds enrolled in preschool. I was allowed to park in the reserved handicapped parking spaces in the school lot. They could carry their children into school or walk with them and hold their hand. I could not. They could run out to their car and back in if they forgot something. I could not. They carried treats into school for their child's birthday. I walked inside to ask for someone to help me or my son had to do it.

When there was an event at school for the moms, I was often asked where my older son was. When I told them he was at home with the nanny, they all thought I was so lucky to have a live in caregiver for my children. They didn't understand it was less of a luxury and more of a necessity for me than other women in town who had help at home.

It was not easy for me to make friends. I think I at minimum made women uncomfortable and in some cases scared them.

My son made friends with the other kids. If they had a playdate I got to hang out with his friend's mother.

I spent some time with Mona who had twins named Katherine and Andrew. When visiting at her house, we spent a good bit of time talking about the usual business of being a mom. She was also curious about the rest of my story. I explained in detail about how I had brain surgery to save my life while I was expecting my son, stayed in the hospital, pregnant and paralyzed for 53 days, and then stayed in a rehab hospital for six weeks to re learn how to walk and take care of myself. Mona asked a lot of questions. She seemed like an intelligent woman who understood everything I said.

Mona and the other mothers at preschool watched me struggle to fit in and get my son through the program.

When our children were four it was time for them to "graduate". They put on an adorable concert in the church affiliated with the preschool. All the parents were there with video cameras. Little four year olds look like miniature college graduates in caps and gowns. The children were called one at a time to walk to get their "diplomas".

Even though it was only preschool, I felt proud of everything my son and my family had accomplished to get to this point in his short life. I was overwhelmed with gratitude for living through a life threatening crisis before he was born and watching him grow up and go to school.

There was a reception after the graduation for the children and the parents to socialize. Many parents were surprised by how quickly the last four years seemed to fly past us. It seemed these kids were just babies and now they were headed to kindergarten.

I sat and sipped tea with Mona. She reminisced briefly about how hectic life had been with twins. I said to her, "I can't believe I'm here watching my son finish preschool after everything that happened."

She said, "Why, what happened?"

For a few minutes I believed I had fooled Mona and everyone else about being disabled the last four years. She seemed to forget I had any issues that made me different.

Chapter 13

The Buffet and All The Other Stuff You Would Never Think Of

I have adapted so well to only using my right hand throughout the day that I assume the habit is as invisible to others as it is to me. I am right handed. My left hand was rendered useless in 1999 by a stroke. It was clenched in a fist and paralyzed. It has slowly regained some function, but I am in such a habit of ignoring it for its uselessness that it has become less useful.

I was recently standing in a buffet line with some close family members at a funeral. Everyone was eager to help me get my food. I asked my niece if she could just lend me a hand and hold the plate for me so I could shovel my food onto it. I explained that that is the part I can't do with only one hand. Another woman in line said "Oh, I never would have thought of that." It hit me then and there that of course we don't think about what it is like to be disabled. I do since it happened to me. I think about people like Christopher Reeve who lived for years with an injury much more disabling than mine. I can manage my own self-care. I live a full life.

Since the funeral, I've been thinking a lot about the other things no one thinks about related to my condition. If I have an itch or bug bite on my right side, my left hand can't usually scratch it. This leads to all sorts of calisthenics whereby I'm rubbing up against a doorway or table edge to scratch. Rather than move my left hand, I end up moving my right arm against my left or other inanimate object.

Likewise, applying lotion or sunscreen to my right side is problematic. Absent someone to help, the cream goes on my leg and I wipe it off with my right arm.

It isn't possible to drive a manual transmission vehicle. Steering a car using only one arm diminishes your safety and ability behind the wheel. I once used a spinner knob to drive which made those turns where you would use the hand over hand turning technique possible and much easier. I put my turn signal on with the same hand I use to steer. Going through a drive through window of any sort poses challenges because they are always configured for left hand use.

I am still working on one handed shoelace tying, but mostly wear shoes without laces.

My right hand is generally occupied by carrying my cane so if I need to open a door for example, I must hold the cane with my left hand and open the door with my right. When walking with the cane, I can't carry much of anything in my left hand.

I have a big head of curly frizzy hair that I used to put in a ponytail.

I haven't quite figured out how to do this one handed.

My title was misleading. This is not a list of ALL the stuff you would never think of, but some that are constant in my life.

Chapter 14
Tribute To An Outstanding Human

There is a man who has received a Valentine card from me every year for the last 20 years even though we never see each other or have any other kind of contact. We "met" on Valentine's Day in 1999 although I have no recollection of it.

I was under general anesthesia when he drilled a hole in my skull, used a saw to cut a piece of it out large enough to access my bleeding brain, cleaned up the hemorrhage, put the piece of my skull back in attaching it with titanium screws, and stapled my skin back together.

It was my stroke of luck on that Valentine's Day when my husband woke up and thought his biggest problem was going to be to figure out where to get me flowers that Dr. B. was the neurosurgeon on call. There is no time to shop for a surgeon when your brain is bleeding.

We learned from the nurses in the neuro intensive care unit that he was about the best neurosurgeon in the area. They said they often see a difference in the outcomes of patients who are lucky enough to have him operate vs. other surgeons which I think is kind of creepy.

I have the dimmest recollection of talking to Dr. B. in the hospital after my surgery. I clearly remember going to his office for a follow up visit months later. He stood in the doorway of his office so he could watch me walk down the hall from the waiting room.

I felt horribly self-conscious as my spastic left arm raised itself over my head of its own accord. I had to hike my hip to clear my braced drop foot to avoid tripping over it. Dr. B. was all smiles.

I sat in his office with my husband as he reviewed the follow up scans of my brain. He was absolutely thrilled to see me walk because he wasn't sure I would be doing as well as I was. He said the hemorrhage had been "extremely large". He couldn't remember performing a craniotomy on another pregnant woman.

When he asked if we had questions, I only had one:

"This is never going to happen again, right?" He said it was extremely unlikely based on how the rest of my brain looked at follow up. The hemorrhage had been caused by a congenital defect in my brain that could have ruptured at any time in my life, or not. He saw no evidence of any other such defects.

There wasn't much call for further office visits once he established I didn't seem to be at further risk of another stroke.

I didn't see Dr. B. again until 2007 when I attended a choral performance at a church my sister had joined before she got married there. Dr. B. was sitting behind me. In his spare time, he had become a deacon in the church.

I asked him if he had been receiving my Valentine cards for the past 8 years as I wasn't sure cards mailed to his office actually reached him.

He told me he did and keeps them in a drawer in his desk and looks forward to getting them every year. I often sent him a photo of the "baby" whose life he saved at the time he saved mine.

When I looked up his address to write his Valentine this year, I read about how he is a leader in the newest cutting edge Cyber Knife brain surgery for brain tumors. In addition to continuing to be a deacon, he also volunteers his time at a local treatment center working with recovering drug addicts in his "spare time".

I have met nurses in the community who have worked with Dr. B. at the hospital. Each and every one of them commented that he is just an outstanding human being.

I wrote the 21st Valentine card to this outstanding human this morning to let him know that 21 years later, I am still grateful for his part in making these years possible.

Chapter 15

Going On Trips With My Brother Is Fun

I have been going on vacations with my older brother who happens to be gay since my husband moved out in 2015. It has been a way to make the best of a bad situation as I was unwilling to stop traveling because I was crippled and alone.

My attorney was instrumental in factoring in a budget for trips for a family of 4 in my separation agreement because that was what we had been spending on vacations in the years leading up to the separation. So my estranged husband was now on the hook for my trips as well as for a necessary travel companion because of my disability. For my first trip without my husband and our sons, I chose a spa hotel in Switzerland because, why not? I always wanted to see Switzerland and the alps. My broken body is always in need of a trip to the spa. So I searched on Google and found a spectacular property in Pontresina, Switzerland. Travel can be a bit dicey when you have a mobility impairment. My brother was willing and able to deal with it for the chance to have a free vacation. He knows what my limitations are and can automatically figure out how to adapt.

My brother was single until this past summer. With the legalization of gay marriage combined with meeting someone suitable, he got married in September.

Until he met his husband, he prowled the dating apps while we traveled. The trip to Pontresina was the first time I traveled without being married. Because my brother and I look like a couple, he goes out of his way to make people understand we are brother and sister just in case anyone is interested in either one of us.

We both are man watchers when we are on tours. When we see someone attractive, we try to figure out which team they are on. Is he for me or you?

There was a handsome concierge at the hotel in Pontresina who appeared to be smitten with me.

My brother made it very clear to him he was *not* my husband, and went on to explain to him that my husband had left me.

The concierge couldn't believe it. He said, "What kind of asshole would leave a beautiful woman like that?" He was embarrassed to use foul language at the front desk of a fancy Swiss hotel. When he heard my husband was paying for everything, he arranged a nice trip up the mountain in St. Moritz with lunch at the top for us.

We made spa appointments and enjoyed luxurious massages and swam in the pool in the atrium with a view of the Swiss Alps. We borrowed the hotel's BMW convertible and drove over the mountains into Italy for some flea market shopping.

The food and service at the hotel was beyond compare. One morning at breakfast, my brother opened the hotel's app on his phone and saw there was a horse show that day in St. Moritz. There were world class equestrians competing at that show which we got to see that day. I couldn't believe I was there.

We had so much fun and worked out the challenges of getting me around safely that we were excited to plan our next adventure when we got home. For all of the fun, I missed being with a romantic partner.

I became involved with a man after that trip and started to plan to take him on my next vacation. I was planning a Rhine River Cruise, and was going to go with my boyfriend. My brother was disappointed, but understood.

After I booked the reservation, my boyfriend relapsed out of sobriety and I told him I couldn't bring him to Europe if he was drinking. I checked with the cruise company to see if I could re book with a different companion due to illness. So I did. I was sad my boyfriend was so sick he couldn't go with me.

Luckily, my brother was free to go on the dates I had reserved for my boyfriend and me.

We made friends on the ship. We made it clear to everyone we were brother and sister. Everyone thought it was so wonderful that we travel together.

We cruised from Basel to Amsterdam where we had a two day extension. My brother encouraged me to change my location on OkCupid to my current location as we traveled so I could chat with men about meeting them. This was a new learning experience for me. I sort of didn't see the point. I had never been promiscuous or had a one night stand in my life.

Cruising down the river didn't make it possible to meet anyone as we were never in one place for long. Until we were in Amsterdam for two full days and nights.

It was there I was emboldened to go on a date at a restaurant with one man, and met another, younger man at our hotel bar and proceeded to hook up with him for my first and only one night stand. I had a false sense of security doing this because my brother was around looking out for me.

For our next trip, I took advantage of a special tour through the alumni association of NYU. We toured the beautiful Amalfi coast in Italy. It was particularly challenging because of my disability in the ancient cobblestone streets. It was well worth the effort. We didn't miss much.

This year we tackled the Canadian Rockies, including two days aboard the Rocky Mountaineer Train. We even did some horseback riding in Lake Louise and Jasper National Park.

I would have been unable to go on these trips by myself. I think I might prefer to travel with a romantic partner, but who knows? Maybe I would ruin a romance by dragging someone around the world with me letting them see me at my most challenged. I am grateful my brother and I get along so well and can spend time traveling   together.

Chapter 16

60 Priceless Hours With Mom

For mother's day, I eschewed traditional gift ideas this year, and instead, insisted that my mother come with me to a world class destination spa for two days. I felt that achieving remission from stage 3 ovarian cancer at her age warranted spending special time together. She is 85 years old, and not very keen on leaving home.

I knew once she was on her way, it would all work out. I was glad she was able to drive herself to my house so we could travel in my car to the spa in Pennsylvania. Before she left her house, she called my sister in North Carolina and told her she wished she was going with her instead because sometimes she needs help, and I am "useless". She was referring to the fact that I have a disability which is something she is still having an awful time getting used to twenty years later.

She arrived at my house at 1:00 on Wednesday and announced that she was "starving". I had made up my mind that for the next 60 hours, I was going to do whatever Mom wanted. When she was done with lunch, I asked if there was anything else I could get for her. She replied, "An ice cream sundae."

"We will stop for ice cream, Mom."

Somehow we got her bag out of her car and into mine. It was too heavy for me to get by myself, so we both lifted it into the trunk.

By the time we both got in the car, I lost track of how many times she'd asked how long it takes to get there. In addition to having hearing loss, Mom isn't the best listener. It is difficult for us to sit in the car for long stretches with our physical challenges.

In true motherly style, Mom asked if I had gas, and wanted to know if I knew how to use my GPS (in the car I've had for five years). I had filled my tank the day before in anticipation of this question. I gave Mom a sort of orientation about where we were going since I had been there on 5 previous occasions. I explained that we could have breakfast and lunch in the bathrobes that would be supplied in our rooms, but would be required to wear clothing of some sort for dinner. Nothing fancy, just clothing.

Mom read every road sign we saw for me. She strolled down more than one memory lane on the way to Pennsylvania. Through the fresh Air Fund in New York City, she went to camp in Sussex, New Jersey as a child from Brooklyn.

We talked about whether we would visit my lake house after we left the spa on Friday. It's about a 40 minute ride. She was concerned we might bother my estranged husband who lives there. I explained that he was not planning to be there until late Friday night. The last time Mom had been to the lake was July 4, 2017. It's about a three hour trip from her house to the lake. We decided to play it by ear for Friday. I really wanted to bring Mom to the cabin. But I was doing whatever she wanted. If she was going to worry about it too much, we could skip it. She ruled out staying over on Friday night because it's too hard for her to sleep in "so many different places." I had thought it might be nice to extend her vacation a little, but it was going to be all about what she wanted.

We stopped at a familiar ice cream stop on the way to the spa for Mom's ice cream sundae. She is very particular about her ice cream so Dairy Queen would not do. The Dairy Bar makes homemade ice cream, and luckily it met with Mom's approval. We were still about 45 minutes from our destination and took advantage of the opportunity to stretch our legs before the last leg of our journey.

The final 45 minute ride was the most scenic, winding up into the mountains on curvy roads through the woods. We stopped at the security gate at the entrance to the spa. Mom was a little impressed they knew we were coming.

She got a little nervous when I parked in front near the valet parking people. "Do we have to take our bags?"

"No, Mom, they will be in our room before we even get there. They have this cool system. It's like magic."

We watched and directed the valet about which bags to take out of my trunk.

The first thing you see when you enter the building is a set of three very large crystal singing bowls set atop a carved, spiral wooden stand. I picked up the soft mallet and showed Mom how to strike the bowls gently to make them sing. The sound was a soothing signal to our bodies to calm down as we arrived.

We stopped at the front desk to check in where Mom made friends with the clerk immediately. She was directed to the ladies room while I registered. I found Mom in the refreshment room down the hall helping herself to some tea. Even though she'd said she wanted to go to the room after visiting the ladies room, she was jumping right into spa life instead. I was so happy to see her figuring out how it worked so quickly. She asked me if my sister had stolen tea bags from the supply when she was there with me on my first visit. The funny thing was my sister had said "Mom is going to have fun stealing those tea bags." The fancy tea bags were a perk of staying at such a luxury destination. We had a good chuckle, and a nice cup of tea and some kind of trifle with dark chocolate spoons.

Mom commented that our room was "far" down the hall as we walked. She loved the luxury appointed room with two queen beds. Our bags were sitting on the luggage racks.

I don't remember how many times Mom had asked me if I was tired on the two hour drive. I wasn't. I was so excited to be having this time with my mother and to be able to do what I could to give her a little getaway.

We looked over the schedule of events for the evening and the next day. There were very few activities that were suitable for us because Mom doesn't drink which ruled out the wine tasting, and neither one of us are active so the hikes and fitness classes were out. All we had to do that evening was show up for dinner for our 6:00 PM reservation.

Mom had brought her bathing suit at my request after asking several times if there was water there. She had looked at the website months ago and had forgotten what it looked like. I explained that there were several hot tubs, a eucalyptus steam room, sauna and indoor pool. Her response was "Oh, I don't know if I can go in the water." We took a wait and see approach. We made light of all the activities we could never do like go mountain biking or go for a power walk. Mom went into the bathroom to check it out. She took inventory of the supplies, reading them out to me as she went: "shower cap, emery board, soap, shoe polish kit, vanity kit." Then she excitedly said, "They do have make up remover towelettes!" I was so relieved that disaster had been averted. I dimly remembered them being there on previous visits.

The meals at the spa were our big activities. The food was delectable, expertly prepared, flavorful and different than our usual fare at home. Of course, it was a luxury to be waited on and not have to clean up. We got an adorable photo taken of us at breakfast in our bathrobes, much like I had done when my sister had been there with me on my first visit.

We enjoyed relaxed, uninterrupted conversation. I shared a lot of stories about my personal life because I know Mom likes that. She likes offering her valuable two cents on everything, too. I was drinking in every minute of having my mother's undivided time and attention. Since she had been sick, we've all recognized the fact that our time with her is not unlimited. This was sort of the point of this trip.

After breakfast on Thursday, our big focus was to be ready for our massage appointments at noon. Mom found a way to worry about what she had to wear to the appointment, as well as what I was wearing. I was going to have less of a traditional massage. I was having Thai yoga massage which requires you to wear loose fitting clothing. I wore workout clothes under my robe which sort of confused Mom. She was still in her nightgown and robe. She was a little concerned about what time lunch would be served until and if we would have time for it after our massages.

She was super impressed by the massage and loved every minute. We had plenty of time for lunch, still in our robes. In fact, Mom stayed in her nightgown that day until it was time to get dressed for dinner. I counted this as a win. I changed into my bathing suit to get in the hot tubs while Mom napped in a chair by the pool. She felt that getting into the water would be "too much work". She noted that the pool was 4 and a half feet deep all the way around, and she is less than five feet tall. There was no lifeguard on duty, and I am "useless". I didn't take too much time in the water because it really was a bit like work after doing so much nothing all day.

We had another day to enjoy great meals, snacks and tea in the Garden Room, and a few lectures there as well. One was about nutrition, the other about sleep. We met the lecturer during the afternoon's nutrition lecture and found her fascinating. She was from Israel, and was a holistic health practitioner, artist, and nutritionist. When we sat for the evening's talk on sleep, it was just the three of us. It was like a private consultation, as well as a friendly visit. She knew where my lake house was, and was familiar with local popular eateries. My mother took the opportunity to share with her as I explained that my estranged husband lives in my lake house which complicates things, and that my husband left me " because he likes to go hiking and I can't hike anymore since I had a stroke." Sure, it's a bit oversimplified, but it conveys the gist of what happened. The speaker gave my mother the "Oh, that's too bad" response she was looking for.

There was a rousing game of bingo after the evening's lecture on sleep. I tried very hard to win, but failed.

We had the option to use the spa's facilities after the noon check out the next day, but we agreed that getting in the water would definitely be too much work. We had made the most of our two days there, taking advantage of what we could. I snuck over to the front desk to check out when Mom was in the bathroom because I knew if she saw how much it cost, it would ruin it for her.

Our bags magically went from our room to my car and my car with more magic appeared at the door when we were ready to leave.

Mom ruled out staying over at the lake house, but wanted me to take her there to see all the changes over the past two years.

On the 30 mile drive, she fretted about whether my husband would be there and if we would bother him. Also, she thought about what if his girlfriend was there when we arrived cooking dinner for him. I glibly replied that it would be cool for his girlfriend to meet his mother in law and it might be nice if she cooked us dinner. Mom was not amused. She admitted that she would not be able to be cordial under those circumstances. I had met his girlfriend and knew I could be cordial, if necessary.

It was a relief when we pulled into the cabin driveway to see no cars. I drove into the new garage to show Mom my husband's new motorcycle. We went in the house and did a quick tour of the new furnishings.

I stopped for another ice cream sundae for Mom on our way back to my house.

We bumped into my estranged husband at my house when we arrived. Mom sat out on the deck with him and got all caught up.

She gave some consideration to staying over at my house before traveling home, but in the end waited for rush hour traffic to abate, then made the trip home by herself.

We had a two day celebration of being alive and well. I'm sure both of us had our patience tried some over the course of so much together time, but it was worth every minute. Life is so uncertain. Grab   it   while   you   can.

Chapter 17
We Were The Misfits

When I was going through one of the toughest challenges in my life, I was surrounded by a group of women who had a unique combination of DNA, surviving catastrophes, living victories, and life experience to support me through it. I think the correct people show up in life for us when we need them most.

Perhaps you have noticed you may attract people who are/have been going through similar experiences to what you are currently dealing with. Support groups may form naturally for us if we keep a look out for them. We should try to join these groups when they appear as they are usually uniquely effective for us in our circumstances. Like attracts like, as the saying goes.

I believe the forces of the Universe conspire to send us the people we need at the moment we need them. It happened to me on more than one occasion.

I had joined a popular weight loss program in 2012. There was a group of women who seemed to gravitate to each other at the meetings. I met each of them over several months, and one day it dawned on me I had become part of this odd little group. Every week, we would sit near each other and catch up with what was going on.

Barbara was trying to lose over a hundred lbs. She had been clean and sober for 25 years so she was no stranger to being able to figure out coping strategies. Each of her daughters had given her enough stress that would have driven your average mother to drink years ago. Her youngest had a child and battled addiction, as well. She had served time in jail. Barbara and her husband ultimately adopted their 8 year old grandson. Her older daughter struggled for years with anorexia. Maryellen was full time caregiver for her severely disabled daughter. She had cerebral palsy and was unable to walk, feed herself or toilet. When her daughter was a toddler, Maryellen had breast cancer at age 37. She had a double mastectomy and reconstruction along with chemo and radiation. Her husband suffered a stroke and went into cardiac arrest after she recovered.

She still had a sense of humor and thought nothing of showing everyone her scars and her new breasts by lifting her shirt in the studio where the meetings were held.

Lisa had lost over 100 lbs. and was constantly adjusting to life as a completely different person. Her marriage crumbled during this process. She had twin teenage daughters.

Sue had battled eating disorders and body image issues on her way to losing 40 lbs. and keeping it off for four years. She had also delivered triplets who were premature and lived the fearful uncertainty of life and death with small babies.

I arrived in the group 13 years after surviving a severe stroke at age 35 during the sixth month of pregnancy. Maryellen was especially tuned in to the fact that I had a disability and was curious and interested in what my abilities were.

I was still walking with a limp, cane and a brace on my foot. My left arm was spastic and nearly nonfunctional.

Over the course of three years, our little group of misfits became very close as we followed each other's struggles.

My own marriage unraveled during this time. Part of the reason was my husband's unwillingness/inability to adapt to life with my disability.

Maryellen was agog when I told her this. She had watched me show up for these meetings for years on my own with a positive attitude and a sense of humor. Having lived with a much more severely disabled person, she was shocked that it seemed hard for anyone to live with me.

This group of misfits seemed uniquely suited to support me through my husband moving out after 28 years of marriage. I think the Universe always sends us the right people.

PART III

The Other Side

Chapter 18

This Is What It's Like Being A Young Woman Who Has Had A Stroke

After profound changes wrought by a devastating stroke when I was 35 years old and 6 months pregnant, my mind, soul and spirit don't feel that different to me.

I went from being vibrant to elderly overnight. I was young, fit and athletic. I woke up on Valentine's Day in 1999 unable to move the left side of my body. Emergency brain surgery stopped the cerebral hemorrhage and saved my life.

I was bed ridden due to paralysis for 53 days after the surgery. I couldn't walk or use my left arm, but I was unchanged inside my head. Family members argued with me when I said I was the same person. I'm sure it's impossible to know what we seem like to other people. But I felt the same. Twenty one years later, my body is still impaired. I limp and carry a cane. I have chronic pain. My left arm and hand are nearly useless.

But I've noticed over the years I still want to BE the same in the world because in my mind I have only changed for the better. I'm resilient and compassionate. I have more patience. I'm tenacious. I want to love and be loved in return. I want attention from men. Passion. Lust. Adventure. Joy. While I am still physically impaired, mostly I am *still* *me*.

Chapter 19

Seduction

The Rehabilitation of My Sex Life.

I t was the activity of daily living no one talked about at the rehabilitation hospital where I spent 6 weeks learning how to live my life again following a severe stroke when I was 35 and 6 months pregnant.

Every day for six weeks, I spent the full day learning how to walk, think, cope, get dressed, cook, and worked on the skills that would be necessary when I returned to driving.

I had psychological counseling to help deal with the postpartum depression made worse by the horrible circumstances of my life. I had a husband and two babies at home and I was in a hospital in a wheelchair.

The occupational therapists tried to teach me how to change a diaper using only my right hand. There was very limited success in this endeavor. My parents brought the baby to the hospital every day so I could nurse him. I used a breast pump to send milk home with them for his bottles.

None of the therapists ever talked to me about rehabilitating my relationship with my husband, including my sex life. It was the topic I dealt with quietly in my own mind, although it was not topmost as I was figuring out how to walk with half of my body left weak and spastic from the stroke.

I imagined everything would be fine when I returned home. I was hospitalized on Valentine's Day and moved to the rehab hospital in April. I went home in a wheelchair in May.

It was a nightmare. I had figured out how to function in the safe confines of a single level hospital with even tile floors, aides to help with everything around the clock, 3 meals prepared for me every day, and help with showering and dressing.

Home was a 2 story house with a sunken living room and a detached garage with steps at both entrances and only 1 handrail on one side at the front door.

My husband was overwhelmed with caring for a 6 week old baby and a two year old, in addition to his adult sized, nearly helpless wife. He was running a business, too.

I continued going to outpatient therapy via senior citizen transportation because I wasn't yet cleared to drive. The subject of my marriage was never discussed at these sessions, either.

I never brought it up because we were in survival mode. It was a struggle to get through every week.

I saw a psychiatrist to treat the depression. He prescribed antidepressants which helped with getting out of bed every day.

It was disturbing to notice that my husband showed zero interest in seeing me naked. Part of the problem was he had been thrust into a caregiver role. Helping me get dressed and undressed was decidedly not sexy.

By October, I was behind the wheel again and walking without assistance.

I continued going to the psychiatrist for medication monitoring and adjustments. One of the best things he did for me was to recommend I find a place to do therapeutic horseback riding to replace the myriad activities I had lost the ability to enjoy.

As the rest of my life was returning to some level of normal, I started to focus on what was missing from my marriage. I told my doctor I was becoming interested in having sex again, but my husband was not.

He was glad to hear I was feeling well enough to be interested in sex. He was a bit mystified by my husband's total lack of interest. He suggested the usual remedies such as date nights and lingerie.

At one session, he asked, "Can't you just seduce him?"

The honest answer was "I don't have the tools." I remembered being able to catch my husband's attention with my sexy body and certain moves before the stroke. Now, my body was broken and I had a movement disorder. I didn't see how I could seduce him now.

I don't remember what is was that made my husband finally come around. I know it took 5 full years.

He seemed to have a laundry list of reasons why he couldn't do it. I was too different. He was traumatized. He was hard wired to only be attracted to a certain "type."

It started out very forced because of the awkwardness of so much time going by and the dramatic changes in my physicality.

What I didn't realize at the outset was that my husband had begun the process of checking out of the marriage. I see it now with the benefit of 20/20 hindsight.

Our sex life continued to be mostly forced. Feeling forced to have sex is not romantic or satisfying for anyone.

I continued to recover slowly and return to more and more "normal" parts of life.

It wasn't until my husband officially checked out of the marriage 16 years later by becoming involved with a woman in another state that my own sex life was resuscitated.

He moved into our vacation home. I found a man near me who found me fascinating and alluring. I still had a movement disorder, but there was no need to seduce him. Scx was satisfying and fun again.

I seem to have no trouble with seduction twenty one year's poststroke. It helps that I am no longer fighting to seduce a man who does not want to be with me.

Chapter 20

Horny, Lonely, Crippled

Many believe sex is better with someone you know and/or love. Despite this, there is still lots of casual hooking up going on. People have various reasons for engaging in this behavior that can also lead to hurt feelings, depression, shame, unwanted pregnancy and sexually transmitted diseases.

Some are simply horny and don't want to be in a committed relationship. Loneliness can also lead people to casual hookups which may bring temporary relief from their sense of isolation. Perhaps oddly, I occasionally hook up with someone not because I'm horny or lonely, but because I am crippled and doing so makes me feel alive and grateful I can still do it.

I was left totally paralyzed on my left side from a stroke during pregnancy when I was 35.I didn't have sex for the next five years until my husband recovered enough from the trauma and my depression lifted enough for me to become interested again. I thought having sex was life affirming and having survived a life threatening ordeal I thought I should be having lots of it. Unfortunately my husband didn't share my enthusiasm. We drifted.

When he thought opening our marriage might help, I reluctantly went along with it because I was willing to do whatever it took to keep the marriage intact. We each started dating other people.

I was not interested in hooking up with anyone just to have sex. I wanted a relationship, too. I met a nice man right away and we had a great time, including lots of sex. He was polyamorous and lived with his girlfriend. So I continued dating new people, too.

Since we weren't monogamous, it occurred to me that I could have sex with anyone I wanted. It looked like an adventure worth trying. Since the stroke, I was about living life all out. I mostly dated around, and only had sex with a few people.

After about two years, I was connecting with someone online who was extremely hot to trot. I realized there was no real reason why I shouldn't just meet him at a hotel near me and try this casual sex thing.

Sure it was a safety gamble. It was also a thrill to feel the freedom and empowerment. Unfortunately, there was some nonconsensual activity with that hookup so I cut ties with the guy.

Being 52 and disabled gave me a sense of being less than desirable sometimes. But I found out this wasn't always the case.

When my boyfriend moved away I connected with a handsome man I had dated a year before just for sex. There wasn't much connection between us otherwise, but the sex was pretty good.

I kept in touch with him even after I met someone else I've been in a relationship with. We have not defined our relationship as exclusive, so occasionally I go to his house for sex just because I can.

I'm not particularly lonely or horny since my boyfriend is great at fulfilling my needs for companionship and sex, but it's important to me to know that another hot guy still wants me and I am able to do this.

I'm here to live life to its fullest while I can. Life is uncertain.

Chapter 21

I Will Let You Think I Need Help Getting Undressed

If That's What Turns You On.

There is a fairly short list of tasks on the "activities of daily living" that I have not been able to adapt to doing with my disability. Over the course of 21 years since I had a severe stroke, I have pretty much figured it all out; showering, driving, cooking, dressing and undressing. There are some major limitations, along with minor ones such as peeling a potato or changing a pillowcase with only one hand which are beyond my abilities.

Most people want to assist me any way they can when they see me struggle with something like zippering up my jacket, and I am usually happy to have the help.

It gets interesting sometimes when a man assumes I will need help getting undressed. Clearly, I have been doing this by myself for 21 years with a disability. But I know men just want to be helpful so I will play along. I also know that for some men, undressing a woman is a major turn on. Maybe better if she's kind of disabled because then she really *needs* the help making them feel more heroic.

Even the guy I have been dating for over a year knows exactly what my abilities are, yet still offers to do things like "help me get out of that sweater". He is just the sweetest, ya know? I have come across more than one such kind soul in my travels.

Sometimes I will exaggerate my lack of coordination and strength because I know it will make a guy feel manly to help me get my clothes off without too much trouble. "Oh, please can you help undo these buttons? I can't get all of them one handed".

It is also fun to make a show of not being able to get in and out of my car gracefully. I can't stand on just my left leg and pivot like normal people do when they get in the car. I sort of fall backwards until my rear end hits the seat, then drag my legs separately the rest of the way. If I'm wearing a dress, I can exaggerate the need to open my legs which makes for a fun show for whomever is holding the car door for me. I can do this when I get out of the car, also, but it looks much more contrived.

I have often thought that having a disability may make me less desirable, but since I have a sense of humor, perhaps the opposite is true.

Chapter 22

I'm Watching You

What I See As A Disabled Woman.

It can't be helped. Everywhere I go I see hordes of people effortlessly doing what I cannot. With exactly half my body affected by a severe stroke 21 years ago, I struggle with a movement disorder.

I'm sure to those with more limiting disabilities, I am the person they are watching wistfully and for that I am grateful. I am able to walk, but not without a struggle. I limp and carry a cane in my functioning right hand. My left hand is nearly useless so if I'm walking, I'm not holding my phone to my ear while drinking a cup of coffee as I open the door to the coffee shop. I see many people do this without thinking. They may even be able to zip up their jacket while doing this, too.

I count myself lucky on a day when I can zip my jacket at all while I'm standing in the house getting ready to go out in the cold. Usually, I can force my left hand to participate enough in this activity to be successful at it.

Since I had the stroke during the sixth month of my second pregnancy, I also saw many mothers carrying one or two children to their cars or the playground where they were able to push them on the swings. Sometimes they held their child's hand while they crossed the street. When my sons were 2 years old and newborn, I was in a wheelchair. I very slowly developed the ability to walk with a cane and a brace on my leg.

In the early days of my recovery, I had to wear orthopedic shoes the brace would fit in. They were usually ugly with Velcro closures since I lacked the fine motor skills to tie shoelaces.

Seeing women strut in high heels bothered me much more in the beginning of my journey than it does now, 21 years later.

I see women crouch in stores to look at products on the bottom shelf. Sometimes in heels.

I see people talking and texting on their phones while they walk through airports carrying suitcases and pulling a roller bag behind them. Maybe they take off their coat at the same time. They might be eating a sandwich or drinking coffee, too. All of this is particularly maddening because I was once one of those people. Until I was 35, I was a dancer and an athlete.

So many years later, I am used to having a movement disorder. I have learned to have gratitude for being alive and able to function. Yet I have not found a way to watch everyone around me move through the world with ease without missing being able to do the same.

Chapter 23

Exactly Half

What I Realized When I Saw A Disturbing Photograph.

The effects from a stroke usually last forever. It's been 21 years since I woke up paralyzed on the left side of my body when I was pregnant.

Spoiler alert: the baby turns 21 this April. Following brain surgery to clean up the hemorrhage that would have killed me if left untreated, the entire left side of my body was completely paralyzed.

During the 53 days I lied in bed in the acute care hospital, pregnant and paralyzed, some movement began to return.

I focused on my fingers intensely and gradually could wiggle them. They were clenched in a fist and my arm was bent and pressing firmly on my big belly. I could pull it away and unfold my fingers with my right hand.

The physical therapists were insistent that I get up and try to walk because I was only 35 and early intervention is critical to stroke recovery. It was scary for everyone because I was pregnant which is not what they were used to working with.

They braced my lifeless left foot and followed me closely as I hobbled around the halls. I couldn't be admitted to a rehab hospital because they weren't equipped to deal with a pregnancy.

Through some miracle I gave birth in the usual way while I was still hemiplegic 6 weeks before the baby was due.

I was moved to a rehabilitation hospital after the birth for intensive physical, occupational and speech therapy while my 2 year old son was home with his father, and the baby stayed with my parents.

For six weeks, I learned how to walk and take care of myself. My thinking was affected in that I had trouble with executive functioning so we worked on that, too.

During that time, I struggled with depression that was caused by being postpartum, organic damage to my brain, and shitty life circumstances. Movement slowly returned, but it was spastic and painful. I was grateful to be able to walk at all. Returning home was a nightmare of an adjustment. It seemed the world had been rearranged in the three months I was in hospitals.

I used a wheelchair at first. We lived in a two story house and my balance was poor. I continued going to outpatient physical therapy for months after my release from the rehab hospital to improve my walking and strength.

It was a slow, painful uphill climb over many years to return to some semblance of a "normal" life. After the first year of recovery, my psychiatrist recommended therapeutic horseback riding as an activity to replace the many sports I could no longer participate in. It was also psychologically helpful in treating the depression.

It's a process that continues to this day, 21 years later.

I've been extremely fortunate to have been able to live my life to the fullest for so many years. I have won 19 ribbons in horse shows since I started to compete in 2014.

I figured out how to continue traveling with my disability. Since I had the stroke in 1999, I have visited Kenya, Costa Rica, Mexico, Switzerland, Germany, France, Italy, the Netherlands, and the Canadian Rockies.

It was on a recent trip to San Francisco to visit my brother when I noticed how odd my face looked in a photograph. At first I couldn't quite name what looked strange.

I studied the picture carefully and realized the left side of my face looked different from the right. It was as if there was a line down the exact center of my face.

The right half was much more animated and the wrinkles were more pronounced due to the greater strength of the muscles there.

It was a bit startling to see this pronounced difference where I had been mostly unaware of the disparity in the strength of the muscles in my face for 21 years.

This jarring realization crystallized and highlighted the fact that I have built a great life with exactly half of my body working properly.

Chapter 24

I usually live in a state of astonishment at being alive.

I don't know if being refined by fire as I was is necessary to achieve this state. I was nearly dead at age 35 from a severe stroke. Living through that experience certainly gave me a renewed appreciation for just being alive.

But in the 21 years since that happened, I suppose I've also become complacent and take much for granted even if I am grateful each day when I can get out of bed.

Living with an awareness that you are doing things others cannot is always helpful. For example, when I am simply driving down the road I can remember it took 7 long months of rehabilitation to even get behind the wheel. I remember that my eyesight is good. My friend had a stroke which affected her eyesight and she's been unable to get her license back.

I am amazed by the complicated ways my brain and body work to operate a car safely in traffic. If you think about it, it truly is astounding.

We often get so caught up in simply trying to stay afloat that we don't "stop to smell the roses." But this is really important. This is part of the key to astonishment.

Keep your eyes open for the miracles that surround us. You can find them in nature, in yourself and other people.

I mentioned the kindness of strangers in my poem. We often rush though our interactions with strangers, but sometimes they go out of their way to be nice. If you take the time to notice kindness, you might be astonished.

Many of us are reeling from the economic downturn caused by the current pandemic. But there are many ways to be rich that don't involve money if we are mindful.

Chapter 25

My Boyfriend Hopes My Husband Still Loves Me

My husband who moved out five years ago brought me 2 dozen red roses last Friday for Valentine's Day. He was taking our sons on vacation on Sunday and will return on Valentine's Day which is why he came a week ahead of time.

He put the flowers in water and left them on my kitchen counter. I asked him how I was supposed to explain them to my boyfriend who was due to come over later that night. With a week of having the house to myself, there's no telling who else may visit through the week and might find it curious there are red roses in my kitchen in advance of Valentine's Day.

Most everyone who knows me is aware my husband and I have been separated for 5 years. They also know Valentine's Day is not just another Hallmark holiday for us.

This year marks the 21st anniversary of the day my husband found me pregnant and paralyzed in the breaking hours of dawn on that freezing morning in February, 1999. He thought his biggest problem when he woke up that day was going to be where to get me flowers.

Instead, he was faced with sending our 2 year old son to the neighbors as I was taken to the hospital in an ambulance. I was 6 months pregnant and had a severe stroke. An emergency craniotomy saved my life as well as the baby's.

Thus began the tradition of making the celebration of Valentine's day about more than cards, candy and flowers. It became a celebration of being lucky to be alive and having friends and family who love me.

This is why my estranged husband still buys me flowers on Valentine's Day. He doesn't want to be my husband, but after knowing each other for 40 years, being married for 28, and having 2 children, we will be like family forever.

Living separately as a "modern family" with each of us being involved with a girlfriend and boyfriend, respectively, often makes for some amusing true facts such as the one that generated the title for this story.

If I am headed to the lake house where my estranged husband lives for my weekend there with my boyfriend, my husband might tell my boyfriend and I to have fun.

He stays in the marital home one or two weekends a month to visit our sons which allows me to enjoy the lake house. My boyfriend finds it amusing to have my husband telling him to have a good time with his wife in the vacation place we shared as husband and wife for so many years. My boyfriend noticed the roses when he arrived that Friday. He said he was glad my husband got them for me as he likely would not.

When we first met, there was still a remote possibility my husband and I might reconcile. He often said he thought it would be a beautiful thing if we found our way back to each other.

In 2 1/2 years, the chances of that happening have gone from slim to none. I don't think my boyfriend thinks reconciliation would be such a beautiful thing anymore.

We were looking at the roses on Sunday when I started to tease him about why my husband got them for me. "He still loves me. He's not over me." He said, "I hope he still loves you. If he doesn't, then he just doesn't get it."

"Doesn't that sound weird for your boyfriend to tell you he hopes your husband still loves you?"

It certainly does sound weird, but the fact of the matter is after a 40 year relationship, we will probably be stuck loving each other for the rest of our lives.

There will be no way to not think of each other on Valentine's Day after living through that traumatic experience on that day in 1999.

Chapter 26
The Tiralo

I think I will miss going to the beach the most until the day I die. Strolling on the water's edge on the sand made firm by the sea water running there and back for eternity, cool water kissing my feet and ankles, squishy sand oozing through my toes, hot sun warming and browning my skin. Turning cartwheels on the firm sand. Running into the water at full speed then diving into an oncoming salty wave. Ducking underwater, dodging dangerous looking big waves. Swimming fast to catch a ride to shore on friendly waves willing to carry me. Being taken by surprise by sneaky powerful waves that knock me down and under, spinning me around until I no longer know which way is up. These are some of the joys of going to the shore.

The beach turned on me when I became disabled. I had a severe stroke when I was 35 and six months pregnant. The baby is now 19 years old. The entire left side of my body became paralyzed. I made a dramatic recovery, but was left with lingering physical deficits that make enjoying the beach nearly impossible. My sense of balance is still very poor. My left foot is paralyzed. I limp and carry a cane. Walking in the sand requires a great deal of assistance. Swimming in the ocean is not possible. I can count the times I have visited the seashore since 1999 on one hand. I remember spending a lazy week on New Jersey's Long Beach Island every summer with friends. They have only invited me once since I became disabled. I think that week was too difficult for me to deal with and too difficult for them to watch because of the new, severe limitations. Where I once jogged around looking sexy in a bikini, I couldn't get into a bathing suit on that trip and wore sneakers with a brace on my leg. I still enjoyed the company on the deck at the house, but was mostly depressed after dragging myself to the beach and being parked in a chair, unable to get up and about. I enjoyed looking at and listening to the surf, but missed the rest of it terribly.

I have had a few more visits to the shore where I was severely limited as far as enjoying the experience. Sometimes I could walk out across the sand on a boardwalk or paved path, or sit on the boardwalk and watch the surf. My husband walked me into the ocean up to my waist once on vacation.

I have had to adapt myriad activities due to being disabled. My family and I went on safari in Kenya with a company that specializes in safari for the disabled. They will provide as much or as little assistance as you need. My husband and son wanted to climb Mt. Kilimanjaro while we were there, and the tour company offered to arrange this trip for me, as well. Climbing was out of the question, but they had access to guides who would carry me the whole way. I was sure this was not the way I wanted to "climb" Mt. Kilimanjaro, especially considering the expense involved. Maybe someday.

Our tour ended in the coastal town of Mombasa at a beautiful beach resort on the Indian Ocean. The water was calm, warm and gorgeous. I felt a strong urge to get in the water. I figured if there were men who could carry me up Mt. Kilimanjaro, there must be someone who could take me in the ocean. The men in my family did not feel confident. I asked our tour directors if they knew of anyone who could carry me in the ocean. They said they would bring me the beach wheelchair, and that my family could take me in that. The chair was called the tiralo.

The weather was perfect the next day when Yvonne dropped the tiralo at our hotel. It was a three wheeled vehicle with fat tires that could roll on the beach and in the water. I sat in it like a toddler in a wagon. There was a handle my 15 and 13 year old sons used to pull me along. They were thrilled to have me as their captive. I was elated to be in their hands. My husband was shooting video of the whole event.

We started at the top of a long hill that led down to the beach. I was given no sign to be ready when I suddenly found myself running down the hill at full speed. It was a thrill, but I still screamed in fear in order to give my sons the desired effect. We laughed a lot in between screams.

We got to the bottom of the hill where there were two cement steps down to the beach. I wanted to stop and engineer my descent. My sons were too quick. They pulled me down the steps. It was a hard hit at the bottom of each. The sand was soft and we continued to run straight into the water. No time to think or test the water. We went directly in. It felt great. It was warm. The tiralo floated on two plastic pontoons. I floated around, going over gentle waves. My husband joined us. I never imagined after that week on Long Beach Island when I was barely able to get around that I would ever be in the ocean with my husband and both sons. The Indian Ocean, no less. It felt like a miracle!

For the most part, the waves were small and gentle and a joy to float over. One strong wave rolled in and flipped the tiralo over with me in it. A pontoon separated from the float. I am not able to swim unaided. The water was too deep for me to stand in.

I briefly went underwater. My 15 year old son swooped into my rescue. He is very strong and sturdy. We started walking toward the beach, but I fell repeatedly due to an inability to gain secure footing in the soft, soaked sandy ocean floor. When he picked me up for the third time, he said "C'mon, Mom, just walk!" I have not been able to walk normally since he was 2 years old. It didn't seem logical that I could take some steps but not be able to continue until we got to the shore. There was no distress, only comedy. I think he felt like the hero he was. I *knew* he would get me safely out of the water.

I don't remember how many times I fell and got back up. I just know we laughed a little harder with each fall. Once ashore, I needed to sit down since walking in the sand required too much effort and assistance. We cobbled the tiralo together so I could sit in it. It was road worthy, but not ocean going. Fortunately, my sons were able to pull me back up the hill to the hotel.

I contacted Yvonne to let her know that the tiralo was broken. I was either brave or foolish enough to want to try it again. She picked it up and said she would have it repaired and returned the next day.

I had the same nerve rattling ride down to the beach the following day. My sons had caught on to the fact that my screams were just for effect so they didn't try anything new to excite me. It turned out to be a beautiful day at the beach with my family. The tiralo held up and carried me through a delightful ride. I now know that adapted enjoyment of pleasures I had enjoyed in the past are better than not doing them at all.

About the Author

Victoria Ponte was born in New York City in 1963. She was raised in New Jersey where she met her husband in 1979. Victoria graduated from NYU in 1985 with a degree in marketing. She was married in 1986 to Mark Leone, an entrepreneur. They had a son in 1997. She had a disabling stroke during her next pregnancy in 1999.

Her marriage ended in 2015.

Her first book, a collection of poetry, was published in June, 2020.

She lives in New Jersey with her two sons and a chihuahua.

For other books by the author visit:

https://www.amazon.com/dp/B08BGD5BP5

Notes

Notes

Notes

Notes

Notes

Notes

Notes

Notes

Notes

Notes

Notes

Notes

Notes

Notes

Made in the USA
Columbia, SC
13 May 2021